*Father,*

*Thank you for the abilities you give us, for the strength and wisdom we gain from training.*

*Be with us as we work that we may do our best. Help us to be encouraging to others in our daily life. Thank you for the people that you have brought into our lives.*

*Bless the athletes, coaches, workout partners and all those who support our training.*

*May the results from our training be a reflection of Your Spirit in our lives.*

*Finally Father, remind us that there is no failure, but only growth in the body, mind and Spirit.*

*Amen*

# Copyright

Cross Training WOD Bible 2.0

586 MORE Workouts To Transform Your Body From Beginner To Beastly!

*First Edition – September 2015*

*Written by P Selter*

Copyright © 2015

All rights reserved.

This book or any portion thereof may not be reproduced or used in any manner whatsoever without the expressed written permission of the publisher except for the use of brief quotation in a book review.

## Disclaimer

The information provided in this book is designed to provide helpful information on the subjects discussed. This book is not meant to be used, nor should it be used, to diagnose or treat any medical condition. For diagnosis or treatment of any medical problem, consult your own physician. The publisher and author are not responsible for any specific health or allergy needs that may require medical supervision and are not liable for any damages or negative consequences from any treatment, action, application or preparation, to any person reading or following the information in this book. References are provided for informational purposes only and do not constitute endorsement of any websites or other sources. Readers should be aware that the websites listed in this book may change.

I recommend consulting a doctor to assess and/or identify any health related issues prior to making any dramatic changes to your diet or exercise regime.

# Contents

Introduction ................................................................ 1

What's New In 2.0? ..................................................... 2

The beauty Of The WOD ............................................ 3

Programming – Because One Size Does NOT Fit All ......... 6

The Power Of The Mind And Taking Consistent Action ... 8

A Quick Refresher On Terminology For Reading &
Following WODs ....................................................... 13

Beginner WODs ........................................................ 15

Bike WODs ............................................................... 22

Bodyweight WODs ................................................... 29

Boxing WODs ........................................................... 39

Dumbbell WODs ...................................................... 63

Jump Rope WODs .................................................... 85

Kettlebell WODs ..................................................... 113

Rowing WODs ........................................................ 123

Running WODs ...................................................... 147

Swimming WODs ................................................... 173

Wall Ball WODs ..................................................... 195

Warmup WODs ..................................................... 221

Conclusion ............................................................. 225

# Introduction

I would like to thank you and congratulate you for purchasing the Cross Training WOD Bible 2.0.

This book is a follow-up to my #1 Best Seller, The Cross Training WOD Bible.

The purpose of this book is to provide you with MORE fantastic info to transform your physique and mindset while having fun doing so!

That's not all this book contains though! You'll also find the Cross Training WOD Bible 2.0 packed with ANOTHER 586 workouts.

These workouts have been broken down into categories based on the content of each workout, these workouts range from beginner workouts that can be performed in the comfort of your own home or backyard to epic endurance workouts utilizing kettlebells, jump ropes, walls balls & more that'll send you to the brink of both mental anguish and physical fatigue.

Thanks again for purchasing this book, I hope it helps you, your friends and your family reach your health and fitness goals!

## What's New In 2.0?

I'm glad you asked!

The Cross Training WOD Bible 2.0 contains 586 NEW workouts! You won't find any of these workouts in the original Cross Training WOD Bible. Kettlebell and bodyweight WODs are fantastic –but I thought it was time to add a tad more variety this time too!

Amidst the plethora of fresh WODs located in this book you'll find many new categories incorporating bikes, jump ropes, dumbbells, rowers, boxing bags and wall balls just to name a few.

## The beauty Of The WOD

Why choose a WOD over a conventional 3, 5 or 7 day workout regime that remains the same week after week?

I understand, if you're new to cross training or are sceptical about the forever changing daily workouts and haven't yet given them a try allow me to explain...

## THE STRUGGLE IS BEAUTIFUL

These workouts are tough, there's no doubt about it.

Why are these workouts tough? Because they're designed for results. You won't find any sissy triceps isolation exercise or pointless movements in the Cross Training WOD Bible – each and every WOD is designed to forge strength and health in both the physical and mental aspects of your life.

## STRESS RELIEF

Swinging kettlebells, giving it your all on the air bike, leaping onto high boxes and hurling your wall ball at the target are all moves requiring an epic amount of exertion – and you're performing these daily.

The stress at your job, the frustration from friends, whatever else you're currently battling through in your life all falls at the wayside while you battle against the clock and yourself to complete your WOD.

**STRUCTURE**

When you get in your car you have a destination in mind and a known path (whether this be a road map or a GPS) to get there. To get results in terms of physical fitness you NEED to have a structured workout. The following 586 workouts are structured based upon the style of workout and equipment you have access to – quite frankly you're spoiled for choice.

Regardless of whether you're a beginner or a time-tested battler there are WODs here for you!

**FITS INTO THE BUSIEST OF SCHEDULES**

So many individuals claim that they "don't have the time to exercise" well, I'm here to the rescue. Dependant on the WOD you choose to perform you'll only need 5 – 15 minutes in most cases!

Everyone has a few spare minutes a day, if you find yourself currently making the excuse that you don't have time to train then I'd recommend waking up 15 minutes earlier, cutting back on 15 minutes of television in the evening – your body and your mind will thank you for it.

Whether you're in your gym, a paddock in the middle of nowhere or a tiny apartment building there is always a suitable, scalable WOD to suit your level of conditioning, the amount of space you have and the arsenal of equipment (or lack thereof) at your disposal.

## ADAPT TO SURVIVE

*"It is not the strongest of the species that survive, nor the most intelligent, but the one most responsive to change"*

Famous, insightful words from Charles Darwin. Why do the same few presses, pull-ups and biceps curls workout after workout, week after week? In order to build both functional strength and an unbreakable mindset to match you need to subject yourself to exercises, workouts, weights and situations that you haven't done before and that you're not quite sure of. It's the unknown and your ability to adapt that will ensure your success. Not to mention variety is the spice of life!

## FORGE A TEAM OF WINNERS

*"Champions come in pairs of two because they battle themselves in perfection"* – Greg Plitt

You can only go so far alone. Many of these workouts are designed to be performed with a partner or a team of multiple members! Forge your own team of winners and perform your WODs with a group of friends... there's many benefits to doing this such as the motivation you'll feed each other, a bit of friendly competition which will force you to lift heavier, train quicker and become better not to mention the relationships you'll form while doing so.

## Programming – Because One Size Does NOT Fit All

You might be completely new to fitness, having never performed a serious workout before... or perhaps you're an elite athlete looking to diversify your workout portfolio.

Either way, no problems whatsoever!

Every WOD is scalable and can easily be adjusted to suit your needs, abilities, strength and current level of conditioning.

### WOD DURATION

Workout durations can be adjusted to cater for inexperienced (shorter duration) or endurance focused athletes (longer duration).

## ROUNDS

Number of rounds can be adjusted to increase or decrease the workload per WOD, this is useful not only based on your current level of physical fitness, but also when time does not permit an exhausting endurance workout.

## REPETITIONS

Repetitions per exercise can be modified based upon the weight of the dumbells, kettlebells, wall ball etc. you're using. Bodyweight exercise repetitions can be decreased to focus more intently on your heavy Olympic lifting movements (this comes down to identifying and programming for your personal goals and focuses).

## SUBSTITUTE EXERCISES

Have a dodgy knee? Can't quite get your chin over the bar on your pull-ups? Don't have enough room to perform a 100m sprint? Substitution is your friend!

For example, if you're unable to perform a 100m sprint why not throw in 30 seconds of high knees?

Do the best you can with what you have.

# The Power Of The Mind And Taking Consistent Action

### *"You can't know where you're going until you know where you've been..."*

Far too many individuals train mindlessly, simply going through the motions of lifting weights and performing cardio while failing to pay attention to detail. It comes to me as no surprise that these are the same people that often fail to see progress, get discouraged, and eventually quit.

On the following pages I'll show you how to do it the right way...

### Disregard the scales and BMI

Before I delve into the methods I use and recommend to track fat loss and muscle gain, I find it imperative to discuss the use of the traditional scale.

### <u>DO NOT BASE YOUR IDEA OF PROGRESS ON WHAT THE SCALES SAY</u>

Weight on the scales, just like the po pular BMI method, is flawed. Muscle mass, fluid retention, time of day, hormones, and a number of other factors can adversely affect the number being displayed to you when you step on the scales.

For example: I've been hovering around the 185lb – 190lb mark. I remember being 185lbs a couple of years ago too... does this mean I haven't bulked or made any progress at all since then? Have I hit an unbreakable plateau?

Of course not.

My body fat has decreased, my fluid retention has decreased and my lean muscle mass has increased... resulting in my total mass clocking in at 190lbs (not to be confused with lean muscle mass, which is my total bodyweight minus my body fat percentage... but we'll get into that later).

According to BMI, body composition is irrelevant — two men, both 230lbs at 5ft 11", would be deemed overweight as lean muscle mass and body fat are not measured on this scale. There are far more accurate methods to measure your progress.

### Take photos and use the mirror

You see yourself on a daily basis, so progress may seem slow or non-existent. This is where taking regular photos comes into play — the mirror doesn't lie.

Choose a location, time of day, and pose and snap the same photo(s) on a weekly or fortnightly basis. When I'm following my cutting diet, I record a video and take several still shots each week, which I find is the most accurate way to gauge progress.

Store these photos in a "Progress" folder on your computer and update them weekly. As you begin to look through and compare your previous week's progress to the current week, you'll often be surprised at just how much your body is changing without you realizing it.

**Take measurements**

Grab a tape measure and take note of your body measurements weekly. I recommend performing these upon waking, as measuring your arms (etc.) post-workout can be inaccurate.

The key to taking successful measurements is to ensure you are measuring in the exact same position every time. Using freckles or placing a mark on your skin is the easiest way to maintain a consistent reference point for measuring.

When measuring, record the following measurements in your training log or in an excel spreadsheet in centimeters:
- Neck circumference
- Shoulder to shoulder (with your arms down by your side)
- Chest (around nipple level, raise your arms to place the tape measure around

your chest and then lower arms before reading measurement)
- Biceps (measure from the peak of the bicep to the thickest portion of the triceps)
- Waist (around your belly button)
- Hips (widest part)
- Quads (choose one spot on your quads and measure this each time)

**Get a caliper**

There are many methods for measuring body fat, some extremely accurate while others are completely inaccurate. The most cost-effective and accurate method in my book is the old caliper test. You can pick up a body fat caliper for $10 online, and it will come with instructions and a chart to help measure your body fat percentage.

**Remain consistent**

Your measurements, photos, training, and nutrition log should be updated consistently. Don't slack off and go through the transformation blindly — have reference points of where you've come from so you can sculpt where you're going.

Seeing progress is THE best motivation to keep the fire alive on your journey.

# A Quick Refresher On Terminology For Reading & Following WODs

**1RM:** Your 1RM is your max lift for one rep

**AMRAP:** As many rounds as possible

**BW**: Body weight

**CLN:** Clean

**C&J:** Clean and jerk

**DL:** Deadlift

**DOMS:** Delayed onset muscle soreness

**DU:** Double under

**EMOM:** Every minute on the minute

**For Time**: Timed workout, perform as quickly as possible and record score.

**KB:** Kettlebell

**OH:** Overhead

**PR:** Personal record

**Rep:** Repetition. One performance of an exercise.

**ROM:** Range of motion.

**Rx'd:** As prescribed, without any adjustments.

**SDHP:** Sumo deadlift high pull

**Set:** A number of repetitions. e.g., 34sets of 8 reps, often seen as 4x8, means you do 8 reps, rest, repeat, rest, repeat, rest, repeat.

**Subbed:** Substituted

**T2B:** Toes to bar. Hang from bar. Bending only at waist raise your toes to touch the bar, slowly lower them and repeat.

**Tabata**: A form of interval training comprised of 20 seconds on, 10 seconds off repeated for 8 rounds.

**TGU:** Turkish get-up

**WOD:** Workout of the day

# Beginner WODs

**Beginner WOD 1**
AMRAP in 10 minutes
5 pull-ups
10 push-ups
15 bodyweight squats

**Beginner WOD 2**
6 rounds for time
6 front squats
3 overhead press
3 deadlifts

**Beginner WOD 3**
10 rounds for time
100m sprint
10 KB swings
10 pull-ups

**Beginner WOD 4**
40-20-10
Burpees
Wall ball shots

**Beginner WOD 5**

4 rounds for time

25 sit-ups

20 walking lunges (10 per leg)

10 push-ups

**Beginner WOD 6**

200m row

20 sit-ups

20 push-ups

20 burpees

**Beginner WOD 7**

21-15-9

Bodyweight squats

Wall ball shots

Burpees

Push-ups

## Beginner WOD 8

For time
40 push-ups
10 bodyweight squats
30 push-ups
20 bodyweight squats
20 push-ups
30 bodyweight squats
10 push-ups
40 bodyweight squats

## Beginner WOD 9

30-20-10-5
5 burpees
10 push-ups
15 bodyweight squats

## Beginner WOD 10

6 rounds
30 second run
30 second push-ups
30 second row
30 second sit-ups
30 second bike
30 second bodyweight squats

**Beginner WOD 11**
AMRAP in 20 minutes
20 sit-ups
15 bodyweight squats
10 push-ups


**Beginner WOD 12**
5 rounds for time
100m sprint
50 jumping jacks


**Beginner WOD 13**
4 rounds
5 minute jog
15 sit-ups
15 push-ups
15 bodyweight squats
5 minute jog

**Beginner WOD 14**

3 rounds
1 pull-up
1 minute sit-ups
2 pull-ups
2 minute push-ups
3 pull-ups
3 minute jog

**Beginner WOD 15**

100 push-ups for time

**Beginner WOD 16**

For time
50 burpees
100 bodyweight squats
200 sit-ups

**Beginner WOD 17**

10 rounds
5 tuck jumps
2 pull-ups
5 push-ups
100m jog

**Beginner WOD 18**

3 rounds for time

10 KB swings

20 walking lunges (10 per leg)

**Beginner WOD 19**

Max reps in 90 seconds per exercise

Push-ups

KB swings

Sit-ups

Walking lunges

**Beginner WOD 20**

4 rounds for time

20 jump rope singles

10 push-ups

3 deadlifts

# Bike WODs

## BIKE WOD 1
3km for time

## BIKE WOD 2
10 minute interval cycling comprised of
30 second work
30 second active recovery (slow ride)

## BIKE WOD 3
8 rounds of cycling comprised of
20 second work
10 second active recovery (slow ride)

## BIKE WOD 4
8 rounds of cycling comprised of
10 second work
20 second active recovery (slow ride)

## BIKE WOD 5
200 calories for time

## BIKE WOD 6
For calories
100-50-25-10-5
Bike
Row

## BIKE WOD 7
5 rounds for time
500m cycle
10 push-ups

## BIKE WOD 8
AMRAP in 20 minutes
Bike for 50 calories
10 burpees
10 sit-ups
10 broad jumps

## BIKE WOD 9
3 rounds for time
200m cycle
100m row
200m cycle
100m run
200m cycle
100 jump rope singles
200m cycle
100 sit-ups

## BIKE WOD 10
10 rounds of
Bike 10 seconds all-out effort
Bike 10 seconds active recovery

## BIKE WOD 11
10 rounds of
Bike 15 seconds all-out effort
Bike 30 seconds active recovery

## BIKE WOD 12
10 rounds of
Bike 20 seconds all-out effort
Bike 40 seconds active recovery

## BIKE WOD 13

10 rounds of

Bike 5 seconds all-out effort

Bike 5 seconds active recovery

## BIKE WOD 14

Bike 10 seconds all-out effort followed by 40 seconds off

Bike 10 seconds all-out effort followed by 30 seconds off

Bike 10 seconds all-out effort followed by 20 seconds off

Bike 10 seconds all-out effort followed by 10 seconds off

Bike 10 seconds all-out effort followed by 20 seconds off

Bike 10 seconds all-out effort followed by 30 seconds off

Bike 10 seconds all-out effort followed by 40 seconds off

Bike 10 seconds all-out effort followed by 30 seconds off

Bike 10 seconds all-out effort followed by 20 seconds off

Bike 10 seconds all-out effort followed by 10 seconds off

## BIKE WOD 15

4 rounds for time

10 push-ups

300m cycle

10 sit-ups

300m cycle

10 squats

300m cycle

10 pull-ups

300m cycle

## BIKE WOD 16

3 rounds

1km cycle as fast as possible

2km cycle recovery ride

## BIKE WOD 17

4 rounds

1km cycle with all-out effort

Rest as necessary between rounds, record your fastest time

**BIKE WOD 18**

5 rounds for time

Cycle for 50 calories

30 second rest

**BIKE WOD 19**

Maintain 70% MHR (max heart rate) for 45 minutes on the bike

**BIKE WOD 20**

10 minutes comprised of

20 seconds all out work

40 second recovery ride

# Bodyweight WODs

## BODYWEIGHT WOD 1
EMOM for 12 minutes
5 burpees
5 broad jumps
6 walking lunges (3 per leg)

## BODYWEIGHT WOD 2
AMRAP in 15 minutes
10 sit-ups
5 burpees
10 mountain climbers

## BODYWEIGHT WOD 3
6 rounds for time
10 pistol squats (5 per leg)
10 box jumps
10 bodyweight squats

## BODYWEIGHT WOD 4
100m sprint
50 pull-ups
50 sit-ups
50 push-ups
50m bear crawl

## BODYWEIGHT WOD 5
AMRAP in 15 minutes
15 burpees
15 push-ups

## BODYWEIGHT WOD 6
AMRAP in 20 minutes
20 walking lunges (10 per leg)
20 air squats
20 burpees

## BODYWEIGHT WOD 7
3 rounds for time
30 broad jumps
10 burpees
30 pull-ups
10 mountain climbers
30 push-ups

## BODYWEIGHT WOD 8
6 rounds
15 jumping jacks
18 walking lunges (9 per leg)
15 push-ups
15 sit-ups
1 minute plank

## BODYWEIGHT WOD 9

8 rounds
10 pistol squats (5 per leg)
1 minute plank
10 jumping jacks

## BODYWEIGHT WOD 10

13 rounds
7 jumping jacks
7 burpees
7 push-ups

## BODYWEIGHT WOD 11

AMRAP in 25 minutes

30 sit-ups

100 flutter kicks

39 sit-ups

100m sprint

50 flutter kicks

50 push-ups

## BODYWEIGHT WOD 12

For time

50 squats

25 diamond push-ups

50 pistol squats

25 fingertip push-ups

50 side lunges

25 knuckle push-ups

50 walking lunges

25 diamond push-ups

## BODYWEIGHT WOD 13

AMRAP in 18 minutes

20 sit-ups

20 toes to bar

20 high knees

20 air squats

20 push-ups

## BODYWEIGHT WOD 14

10 rounds for time

10 burpees

10 sit ups

10 jumping jacks

10 air squats

50m dash

## BODYWEIGHT WOD 15

Tabata (8 intervals – 20 seconds work – 10 seconds rest)
Air squats
Push-ups
Sit-ups
Jumping jacks

## BODYWEIGHT WOD 16

4 rounds for time
10 burpees
20 squats
30 sit-ups
40 walking lunges (20 per leg)

## BODYWEIGHT WOD 17

3 rounds for time
50 burpees
10 pull-ups
50 diamond push-ups
5 tuck jumps

## BODYWEIGHT WOD 18

EMOM for 12 minutes

3 burpees

4 flutterkicks

5 push-ups

5 sit-ups

## BODYWEIGHT WOD 19

For time

40 walking lunges

80 squats

10 push-ups

60 squats

20 wide push-ups

40 squats

30 diamond push-ups

20 squats

## BODYWEIGHT WOD 20

3 rounds

Max push-ups in 2 minutes

Max sit-ups in 2 minutes

Max mountain climbers in 2 minutes

Max squats in 2 minutes

## BODYWEIGHT WOD 21
5 rounds for time
15 box jumps
30 push-ups
45 sit-ups
5 pistol squats


## BODYWEIGHT WOD 22
21-15-9 for time
Box jumps
Pistol squats
Diamond push-ups

## BODYWEIGHT WOD 23
50-40-30-20-10-5 for time
Pull-ups
Bodyweight dips
Walking lunges (per leg)

## BODYWEIGHT WOD 24
50-40-30-20-10 reps
Squat jumps
Jump rope singles
Sit-ups

## BODYWEIGHT WOD 25

EMOM for 14 minutes

3 pull-ups

3 sit-ups

3 squat jumps

3 diamond push-ups

## BODYWEIGHT WOD 26

For time

21 pull-ups

50 squats

21 toes to bar

18 pull-ups

50 squats

18 squat jumps

15 walking lunges (per leg)

50 squats

15 toes to bar

12 pull-ups

## BODYWEIGHT WOD 27

EMOM for 15 minutes
5 air squats
6 lunges (3 per leg)
5 mountain climbers

## BODYWEIGHT WOD 28

For time (partition as necessary)
100 pull-ups
100 push-ups
100 sit-ups
100 mountain climbers

## BODYWEIGHT WOD 29

3 rounds for time
20 toes to bar
20 sit-ups
50 mountain climbers
50 squat jumps

## BODYWEIGHT WOD 30

8 rounds for time
20 diamond push-ups
40 sit-ups
20 wide push-ups
20 box jumps
20 jumping jacks

# Boxing WODs

## BOXING WOD 1

Skipping 30 seconds 3 sets

Speed Bag 2 minutes

Squat Thrusts 3 sets 10 reps

Heavy bag or Mitt jabs x 10

Repeat for 4 rounds

## BOXING WOD 2

Combo Shoulder Raise (with dumbbells) 4 sets 20 reps

Sit-up 4 sets 20 reps

Shadow boxing 2 mins

Single arm neutral grip dumbbell row 4 sets 10 reps each arm

Shadow boxing 2 mins

Standing dumbbell biceps curl 3 sets 10 reps

Shadow Boxing 2 mins

## BOXING WOD 3
Lateral Leap and Hop 3 sets 10 reps
Heavy Bag or mitt work - Crosses x 10
Heavy bag or mitt work – Uppercuts 10 reps
Lying leg curls 3 sets of 10 reps
Heavy bag or mitt work – Jab 10 reps
Heavy bag or mitt work – Hook 10 reps
Repeat x 2

## BOXING WOD 4
Dumbbell Bench Press 4 sets 10 reps
Bodyweight Dip 3 sets 10 reps
Speed Bag 1 min 3 reps
Skipping 30 secs 3 reps
Lunge Thrusts 4 sets 20 reps
Sit-ups 4 sets 20 reps

## BOXING WOD 5
Barbell Deadlift 4 sets 10 reps
Wide Grip Lat Pull Down 4 sets 10 reps
Shadow Boxing 2 mins
Heavy Bag or Mitt Work – Jab 10 reps
Heavy Bag or Mitt Work – Hook 10 reps
Heavy Bag or Mitt Work – Cross 10 reps

## BOXING WOD 6

Heavy Bag or Mitt work – Boxing combinations Jab, Hook, Cross 30 secs

Sit-ups 30 secs

Squat Jumps 30secs

Repeat x 10

## BOXING WOD 7

Push Ups 50 reps

Situps 50 reps

Speed Bag 3 mins

Heavy Bag/Mitts – combination punches 3 mins

Repeat for 5 rounds with 1 min rest in between

## BOXING WOD 8

100m sprint

Push ups 3 sets 20 reps

Sit ups 3 sets 20 reps

100m sprint

Squat thrusts 3 sets 20 reps

Speed Bag 1 min 3 reps

5km run

## BOXING WOD 9
Air Box Jab/Cross 40 sets (1,2,1,2 etc)
Flutter kicks 15 reps
Air Box Jab/Cross 40 sets
Burpee 15 reps
200m sprint
Repeat for 2 rounds

## BOXING WOD 10
Decreasing set of 50-40-30-20-10
Skipping (Double unders)
Sit ups

## BOXING WOD 11
Shadow Boxing 2 mins
Squat Thrusts 2 sets 10 reps
Kettle Bell Snatches 2 sets 10 reps
Sit ups 2 sets 30 reps
Speed Boxing 1 min 3 reps
Repeat for 4 rounds

## BOXING WOD 12

Single arm kettle bell swing 10 reps each arm 2 sets

Burpees 4 sets 10 reps

Heavy bag or Mitt work – Jab/Uppercut/Cross combination for 10 reps

Kettlebell Squat Swing 2 sets 10 reps

Squat Thrusts 4 sets 10 reps

Heavy Bag or Mitt work – Combination for 10 reps

## BOXING WOD 13

5km run

Speed bag 1 min 3 reps (30 sec rest in between)

Skipping 3 mins

Speed bag 1 min 3 reps

Repeat 2 rounds

## BOXING WOD 14

Knees to elbows pull up bar repeat to fail x 3 sets

Squats 3 sets 20 reps

Plank 30 secs

Burpees 3 sets 20 reps

Shadow boxing (gloves on) 2 mins, 1 min rest, repeat x 5 sets

Plank 30 secs

## BOXING WOD 15
100m sprint
Speed bag 30 secs
100m sprint
Burpees 20 reps
100m sprint
Speed bag 30 secs
100m sprint
Push ups 20 reps
Repeat for 3 rounds

## BOXING WOD 16
Chin ups/Pull ups 3 sets 10 reps
Squats 3 sets 10 reps
Shoulder press 3 sets 10 reps
Walking Lunges 3 sets 10 reps

## BOXING WOD 17
Air box – Jab/Cross repeating 2 sets
Skipping – 20 reps each of high knee, single jump, double jump, figure eight
Push Ups 2 sets 20 reps
Repeat for 5 rounds

## BOXING WOD 18

Crunches 3 sets 20 reps

Heavy Bag or Mitt work – Jab 10 reps

Heavy Bag or Mitt work – Cross 10 reps

Speed bag – 2 mins

Crunches 3 sets 20 reps

Burpees 3 sets 20 reps

## BOXING WOD 19

Skipping 1 min

Air boxing: – Left, left, right, duck 12 reps

Upper cuts 12 reps

Left, Right punches 12 reps

Crunches 20 reps

Side lunges 10 reps each side

Donkey kicks 10 reps each side

Left, left, right, duck 12 reps

Upper cuts 12 reps

Left, Right punches 12 reps

Squats 10 reps

Back lunges 10 reps each side

Push up 10 reps

Skipping 1 min

## BOXING WOD 20

Round 1:

Straight punches 20 reps

Burpees 10 reps

Bicycle abs 20 reps

Round 2:

Hooks 20 reps

Push ups 20 reps

Dolphin plank 20 sec

Round 3:

Uppercuts 20 reps

Dips 10 reps

Sit ups 30 reps

Repeat for 3 rounds and cooldown with 2 mins skipping

**BOXING WOD 21**

(With heavy bag/punchbag)

Low kick right leg 5 reps

High kick right leg 5 reps

Low kick left leg 5 reps

High kick left leg 5 reps

Straight Punches 20 reps

Left Hook 5 reps

Right Hook 5 reps

Knee strike 5 reps

Repeat for 5 rounds with 30 sec rest between each round

**BOXING WOD 22**

Clapping push up 2 sets 10 reps

Explosive Box jumps 2 sets 20 reps

Squats 2 sets 30 reps

Medicine ball lunges 20 reps each leg

Medicine ball step to press (with step up) 20 reps each leg

One arm dumbbell row 15 reps each arm

Ab roller 15 reps from knee, or 50 crunches if no equipment

Chin ups 2 sets 8 reps

3 rounds of heavy bag work – combination of punches 30 secs each round

3 rounds speed bag – 30 sec each round

Finish with 2 mins shadow boxing

## BOXING WOD 23

Skipping 3 mins

Air boxing – jab, cross, jab, bob and weave 10 reps each side

Push ups starting in Plank position 10 reps

Air Box – jab, cross, jab, cover 10 reps each side

Push ups as before 10 reps

Air Box – jab, cross, jab, bob and weave 10 reps each side

Bicycle crunches 20 reps

Air box – jab, cross, upper and cover

Bicycle crunches 20 reps

Finish with criss-cross skipping 3 mins

## BOXING WOD 24

5-10 min warm up skipping

High speed jab and crosses 20 secs

Squats 10 secs

Repeat for 8 rounds

Upper cuts 20 secs

Lunges 10 secs

Repeat for 8 cycles

5 min Cool down skipping and stretch

## BOXING WOD 25

Fast and loose straight punches 1 min

Knuckle press ups 10 reps

Plyometric press up 6 reps

Fast and loose combination punches 1 min

Squat and hold 30 secs

Frog jump 10 reps

Repeat for 5 rounds

## BOXING WOD 26

Heavy Bag Work: Round 1

Straight jabs 60 reps

Jab to body 30 reps

High double jab 30 reps

Jab/Cross combo 60 reps

Round 2:

Cross 60 reps

Cross to body 30 reps

Jab/Cross combo 3 reps

Lead hooks 60 reps

Round 3:

Rear hook 60 reps

Jab/Cross/Hook combo 30 reps

Lead hook to body 30 reps

Rear hook to body 30 reps

**BOXING WOD 27**

Burpees 20 reps

Mountain climbers 20 reps

Straight air punches 30 secs

Front air kicks 30 secs

Squat jumps 20 reps

Alternating side air kicks 30 secs

Repeat for 3 rounds

**BOXING WOD 28**

Jumping jacks 100 reps

Push ups 10 reps

Squat jumps 10 reps

Tricep dips 20 reps

High knees (fast) 30 reps

Bicycle crunches 50 reps

Burpees 15 reps

Push ups 20 reps

Curtsy Lunges 15 reps each side

Wide stance squats 40 reps

Repeat as many times as possible in 30 mins

## BOXING WOD 29

8 jabs, 8 uppercuts, repeat for 20 secs

Hook and Weave 20 secs

High knee jump rope 20 secs

Roundhouse kicks, 4 each leg and repeat for 20 secs

Repeat for 8 rounds

## BOXING WOD 30

Shadow boxing 5 mins with double squat every 30 secs

Push ups 10 reps

Sit ups 20 reps

Repeat 5 rounds

## BOXING WOD 31

1 minute for each:

Jump rope

Burpees

Jump rope

Press ups

Jump rope

Sit ups

Jump rope

Squats/Squat jumps

Jump rope

Spiderman plank

Repeat for 4 rounds with 1 min rest in between

## BOXING WOD 32

Box non-stop for the duration of an upbeat song

Rest for 1 minute

Repeat for 5 songs

## BOXING WOD 33

Skipping 3 minutes
1 minute of each:
Left jab/Right cross
Squat jumps
Basic 1-2 punch
Push ups
Burpees
Right jab/Left cross
Lunge jumps
Basic 1-2 punch
Bicycle crunches
Plank


## BOXING WOD 34

30 secs per exercise as fast as you can:
Punch to front
Punch to side (alternate)
Uppercuts
Punch to sky
Double punch to front
Double punch to sky
Repeat for 3 rounds resting 1 min between rounds

**BOXING WOD 35**

Push ups 50 reps

Squat jumps 50 reps

Sit ups 50 reps

Lunges 50 reps

Tricep dips 50 reps

Back extensions 50 reps

**BOXING WOD 36**

High knees 40 reps

Push ups 20 reps

"Rocky" reverse crunches 20 reps

Shadow boxing 5 mins

**BOXING WOD 37**

Sit ups 20 reps

Sit up and punch 20 reps

Sit up and touch toes 20 reps

Oblique sit up 20 reps

Ab cycle 20 reps

Back extensions 20 reps

Spiderman plank 20 secs

## BOXING WOD 38

Jog 1 min

Shadow box 3 mins

Jog 1 min

Boxing round 1 (1 min jab, hook, uppercut, 2 min throw combos)

Jog 1 min

Boxing round 2 (3 mins all combos)

Jog 1 min

Boxing round 3 (3 mins all combos)

Jog 1 min

Jump rope 3 mins

Jog 1 min

Shadow box 3 mins

## BOXING WOD 39

Jabs/Crosses/Push-ups 3 sets 10 reps

Jab crosses/Squats/Squat jumps 3 sets 10 reps

10 round kicks each leg 3 reps

Hook punches alternate arms / Burpees 3 sets 10 reps

## BOXING WOD 40

Push ups 25 reps

Pull ups 25 reps

Squat Jumps 25 reps

25 Burpees 25 reps

Air box – cross/jab/hook combo 3 mins

Repeat for 4 rounds with 1 min rest between rounds

## BOXING WOD 41

Run 100m
30 uppercut punches on heavy bag
Run 100m
30 hooks on pads
Repeat for 12 rounds

## BOXING WOD 42

30 uppercut punches on heavy bag
30 flutter kicks
30 side hook punches on heavy bag
30 sit-ups
100m run
Repeat for 7 rounds

## BOXING WOD 43

40 straight punches
10 uppercuts
10 side hooks
30 seconds rest
40 straight punches
20 sit-ups
30 second plank
Repeat for 7 rounds

## BOXING WOD 44

1 minute on, 1 minute off of the following:
30 straight punches
10 sit-ups
30 side hooks
10 sit-ups
30 uppercuts
Repeat for 20 minutes

## BOXING WOD 45

Complete 10 rounds as quick as possible of:
20 air squats
20 push-ups
20 straight punches
20 sit-ups
20 walking lunges
20 box jumps

## BOXING WOD 46

7 rounds of:
10 double-unders
1 minute shadow boxing
Run 200m
10 sit-ups
10 air squats

## BOXING WOD 47

As many rounds as possible in 10 minutes:
12 straight punches
12 burpees
12 sit-ups
12 jumping jacks
12 push-ups

## BOXING WOD 48

Complete the following as fast as possible:
50 double-unders
50 sit-ups
50 box jumps
20 straight punches
20 uppercuts
20 side hooks
20 mountain climbers
20 burpees
20 jumping jacks

## BOXING WOD 49

Complete 5 rounds as quick as possible of:
20 air squats
20 push-ups
20 straight punches
50 double-unders
50 sit-ups
50 box jumps

## BOXING WOD 50

3 rounds of:

Shadow Boxing 1 min

Squat Thrusts 20 reps

Kettle Bell Snatches 20 reps

Sit ups 60 reps

# Dumbbell WODs

## DB WOD 1
21-15-9
DB thrusters
Burpees
100m sprint

## DB WOD 2
300m sprint
21 DB deadlifts

## DB WOD 3
100 DB push press
20 jump rope singles
10 HSPU
20 DB thrusters

## DB WOD 4
EMOM for 15 minutes
10 DB swings
20 DB push press

**DB WOD 5**

6 rounds for time
10 push-ups
15 DB hang squat cleans
15 walking lunges (per leg)
15 DB deadlifts

**DB WOD 6**

For time
100 DB hang squat clean thrusters
100 burpee broad jumps

**DB WOD 7**

AMRAP in 12 minutes
10 DB push ups
10 sit-ups (holding DB)
10 DB snatch (per arm)

**DB WOD 8**

For time
100 air squats
100 DB squats
100 DB push-ups
10 burpees
10 broad jumps

## DB WOD 9

Start a clock:

Run for 5 minutes at a moderate pace on the treadmill.

At minute 6 perform max snatches in 2 minutes alternating arms with the dumbbell.

At minute 9 perform max KB swings w/dumbbell in 1 minute

At minute 11 perform max front squats holding the same dumbbell for 2 minutes

At minute 14 perform max burpees for 1 minute

## DB WOD 10

AMRAP in 12 minutes

14 bodyweight dips

14 walking lunges (per leg)

14 DB shoulder press

## DB WOD 11

5 Rounds for time

10 mountain climbers

7 DB squat cleans

4 DB deadlifts

**DB WOD 12**
EMOM for 10 minutes
10 DB push press
2 burpees

**DB WOD 13**
For time
100 DB deadlifts

**DB WOD 14**
40-20-10-5
DB Thrusters
Walking lunges holding DB
Burpees

**DB WOD 15**
EMOM for 15 mins
3 DB squats
5 push ups
7 DB thrusters
9 walking DB lunges (per leg)

## DB WOD 16
For time
400m sprint
40 DB one arm snatch (right)
400m sprint
40 DB one arm snatch (left)
400m sprint

## DB WOD 17
80 jump rope singles
10 DB snatches (per arm)
10 DB thrusters
10 Turkish get ups
100m sprint

## DB WOD 18
AMRAP in 5 minutes
5 DB shoulder press
5 pull-ups (holding DB)
5 dips (holding DB)

**DB WOD 19**
5 rounds for time
200m sprint
35 dumbbell squats
10 toes to bar
35 DB shoulder press

**DB WOD 20**
AMRAP in 20 minutes
400m sprint
40 DB thrusters

**DB WOD 21**
9 rounds for time
10 DB snatches (per arm)
100m sprint

**DB WOD 22**
EMOM for 17 minutes
7 DB thrusters
7 DB lunges

## DB WOD 23
3 rounds for time
200m sprint
30 DB clean and press
20 DB squats
300m sprint

## DB WOD 24
3 rounds for time
18 DB swings
18 sit-ups

## DB WOD 25
30-25-20-15-10-5-1
Dumbbell shoulder press
Jump rope singles
Burpees

## DB WOD 26
21-15-9
DB hang cleans
Pull-ups

**DB WOD 27**

For time

21-15-9

DB swing single arm

DB single arm push press

Mountain climbers

**DB WOD 28**

EMOM for 20 minutes
5 DB thrusters

**DB WOD 29**

3 rounds for time

25 DB deadlift

20 DB swings

15 DB push press

100 mountain climbers

**DB WOD 30**

For time

100m sprint

20 DB walking lunges (per leg)

20 push-ups

20 sit-ups

100m sprint

## DB WOD 31
10 rounds for time
15 DB goblet squats
15 DB floor press

## DB WOD 32
EMOM for 20 minutes
10 bodyweight squats
10 pull-ups
10 DB floor press
10 DB goblet squats

## DB WOD 33
5 rounds
40 seconds per exercise
DB push press
DB one arm row
DB front squat
400m sprint

## DB WOD 34
AMRAP in 12 minutes
400m sprint
4 DB deadlifts

## DB WOD 35
For time
12-10-8-6-4-2
DB one arm row (per arm)
DB deadlift
DB thrusters

## DB WOD 36
For Time
21-15-9-6-3-1
DB hang clean
DB push up
DB snatch

## DB WOD 37
10-5-1
DB deadlift
DB floor press
DB walking lunges (per leg)

## DB WOD 38
AMRAP in 15 minutes
20 burpees
20 DB thrusters

**DB WOD 39**

AMRAP in 17 minutes

10 DB power cleans

10 Turkish get-ups

**DB WOD 40**

5 rounds for Time

8 pull-ups

8 DB goblet squats

8 sit-ups

**DB WOD 41**

As many rounds as possible (3 minutes per round)

1 minute DB push press

1 minute DB walking lunges

1 minute DB deadlifts

**DB WOD 42**

For time

100 DB floor press

100 push-ups

100 bodyweight squats

100 DB walking lunges

**DB WOD 43**

Tabata each exercise

DB front squat

DB swings

DB thruster

**DB WOD 44**

AMRAP in 21 minutes

10 burpees

10 DB thrusters

10 DB front squats

**DB WOD 45**

For time

21-15-9

HSPU

DB renegade row

100m sprint

Floor press

Push-ups

**DB WOD 46**

4 rounds for time
8 DB swings
8 push-ups
8 Turkish get-ups
80m dash

**DB WOD 47**

For time
25 DB thrusters
25 DB Ground-to-Overhead
25 DB renegade rows
25 DB push press
25 DB front squats

**DB WOD 48**

EMOM for 21 minutes
12 DB goblet squats
12 push-ups
12 DB renegade rows

**DB WOD 49**

7 rounds for time
12 DB deadlifts
12 burpees
100m sprint

**DB WOD 50**

EMOM for 15 minutes
4 DB push-ups
4 DB floor press
4 dips

**DB WOD 51**

For Time:
20-18-16-14-12-10-8-6-4-2-1
Tuck jumps
DB walking lunges
DB squats
DB thrusters
DB push press

## DB WOD 52
AMRAP in 20 minutes
5 burpees
10 weighted sit-ups (holding DB)
15 DB goblet squats

## DB WOD 53
For time
50 jump rope singles
50 burpees
50 DB clean and press
50 DB walking lunges (per leg)
50m dash

## DB WOD 54
For time
100 weighted push-ups (holding DB)
100 weighted sit-ups (holding DB)
100 DB front squats

**DB WOD 55**
10 min AMRAP
5 Tuck Jumps
5 Plyo Pushups
5 Jump Squats
30 Sec Plank

**DB WOD 56**
20 sec Work 10 sec Rest for 8 Sets
In order
DB push press
DB walking lunges
Jump rope singles
DB deadlifts

**DB WOD 57**
5 Rounds for time
50 DB floor press
100m sprint
50 DB goblet squats

## DB WOD 58
Max DB squats in 1 minute
30 sec rest
Max DB push-ups in 1 minute
30 sec rest
Max DB walking lunges in 1 minute
30 sec rest
Max DB push press in 1 minute
30 sec rest
Max sit-ups (holding DB) in 1 minute

## DB WOD 59
For time
21-15-9-4-3-2-1
DB walking lunges (per leg)
Double-unders
Box jumps
DB floor press

## DB WOD 60
50 Jump rope singles
9 DB thrusters
9 DB push press
18 DB walking lunges (9 per leg)

**DB WOD 61**

For time

50m sprint

25 weighted push-ups (with DB on back)

50 sit-ups

25 DB front squats

50 DB renegade rows

**DB WOD 62**

AMRAP in 15 minutes

5 push-ups

10 DB shoulder press

15 DB squats

10 mountain climbers

**DB WOD 63**

3 rounds for time

2 minutes jump rope singles

5 weighted push-ups (with DB on back)

25 DB floor press

25 DB renegade rows

25 DB cleans

## DB WOD 64
For time
100 weighted dips (with DB strapped to waist)
100 weighted pull-ups (with DB strapped to waist)
Rest as necessary

## DB WOD 65
3 Rounds for time
400m sprint
30 DB thrusters
30 DB floor press

## DB WOD 66
AMRAP in 16 minutes
10 DB thrusters
10 Burpees
10 DB push-ups
10 Burpees
10 DB renegade rows

## DB WOD 67
EMOM for 10 minutes
5 deadlifts
5 push presses
5 DB goblet squats
50 DB Russian twists (holding DB while rotating side to side)

## DB WOD 68
For time
50 DB thrusters
100 push-ups
50 DB swings

## DB WOD 69
10-9-8-7-6-5-4-3-2-1
DB walking lunges
DB renegade rows
Turkish get-up
DB shoulder press

**DB WOD 70**

AMRAP in 7 minutes

10 DB floor press

10 DB push press

20 mountain climbers

10 DB walking lunges (5 per leg)

10 DB front squats

# Jump Rope WODs

**Beginner Jump Rope WOD 1**
AMRAP in 10 minutes
20 singles
10 push-ups
5 double-unders
10 bodyweight squats

**Beginner Jump Rope WOD 2**
For time
500 singles

**Beginner Jump Rope WOD 3**
AMRAP in 20 minutes
50 singles
5 pull-ups
50 singles
5 push-ups
50 singles
5 bodyweight squats

**Beginner Jump Rope WOD 4**
For time
20 singles
20 box jumps
20 push-ups
20 toes to bar
20 singles
5 double-unders
200m row

**Beginner Jump Rope WOD 5**
For time
 20 jump rope singles
40 wall ball shots
60 burpees
80 jump rope singles
500m sprint

**Beginner Jump Rope WOD 6**
4 rounds for time
40 jump rope singles
10 thrusters
20 box jumps
30 sit-ups
40 jump rope singles

**Jump Rope WOD 1**

3 rounds
50 jump rope singles
10 clean & jerks
50 double-unders

**Jump Rope WOD 2**

For time
10 pull-ups
10 jump rope singles
10 push-ups
10 jump rope singles
20 pull-ups
30 jump rope singles
40 push-ups
50 jump rope singles

**Jump Rope WOD 3**

5 rounds
10 KB Turkish get-up
20 jump rope singles
30x flutter kicks
40 double-unders

**Jump Rope WOD 4**
For time
 50 double-unders
10 burpees
40 double-unders
20 sit-ups
30 double-unders
30 jumping jacks
20 double-unders
40 walking lunges (20 per leg)
10 double-unders
50 pull-ups

**Jump Rope WOD 5**
4 rounds
500m sprint
4 pull-ups
40 jump rope singles

**Jump Rope WOD 6**
5 rounds
 50-40-30-20-10
Jump rope singles
Thrusters
Double-unders

**Jump Rope WOD 7**
For time
50 double unders
10 handstand push-ups
40 double unders
8 handstand push-ups
30 double unders
6 handstand push-ups
20 double unders
4 handstand push-ups
10 double unders
2 handstand push-ups

**Jump Rope WOD 8**
8 rounds
150m row
20 wall ball shots
50 jump rope singles
25 double-unders

**Jump Rope WOD 9**
10 rounds for time
5 power cleans
10 pull-ups
15 double-unders

## Jump Rope WOD 10
For time
20 double-unders
5 pull-ups
6 push-ups
7 pull-ups
8 squats
9 pull-ups
100 jump rope singles

## Jump Rope WOD 11
20 pull-ups
10 double-unders
20 pull-ups
10 deadlifts
20 pull-ups
10 split squats
10 double-unders
20 pull-ups
10 burpees
20 pull-ups
10 toes to bar
20 pull-ups
10 double-unders

## Jump Rope WOD 12

For time
6 double-unders
100m row
6 double-unders
20 handstand push-ups
6 double-unders
30 ring dips
6 double-unders
30 push-ups
6 double-unders
30 sit-ups
6 double-unders

## Jump Rope WOD 13

3 rounds
20 mountain climbers
30 sit-ups
1 minute jump rope singles
10 double-unders
1 minute jump rope singles
10 double-unders
30 sit-ups

## Jump Rope WOD 14

90 seconds per exercise, rotate for 3 rounds
Burpees
Jump rope singles
Push-ups
Jump rope singles
Pull-ups
Jump rope singles
Squats

## Jump Rope WOD 15

5 rounds
15 double-unders
15 pull-ups
15 squats
15 box jumps
15 push-ups
15 double-unders

**Jump Rope WOD 16**

For time
Row 70 calories
10 double-unders
Row 70 calories
20 double-unders
Row 35 calories
30 double-unders
Row 35 calories

**Jump Rope WOD 17**

2 rounds for time
21 double-unders
10 burpees
10 broad jumps
10 Pull-ups
10 goblet squats
10 box jumps
10 jump rope singles

**Jump Rope WOD 18**

AMRAP in 12 minutes
5 thrusters
5 pull-ups
10 double-unders

**Jump Rope WOD 19**

3 rounds for time
24 double-unders
24 KB swings
24 jump rope singles
24 mountain climbers

**Jump Rope WOD 20**

AMRAP in 20 minutes
200m sprint
10 HSPU
10 jump rope singles
200 double-unders

**Jump Rope WOD 21**

3 rounds
 20 pistol squats
20 double-unders
20 push-ups
20 toes to bar

## Jump Rope WOD 22

AMRAP in 17 minutes

50m swim

50m sprint

50 jump rope singles

30 second plank

50 double-unders

## Jump Rope WOD 23

3 rounds

21-15-9-5-1

Jump rope singles

Wall ball shots

Sit-ups

Double-unders

## Jump Rope WOD 24

6 rounds for time

5 double-unders

5 KB clean & press

5 DB push press

5 jump rope singles

5 KB swings

5 deadlifts

**Jump Rope WOD 25**
AMRAP in 10 minutes
15 Double-unders
15 Handstand push-ups

**Jump Rope WOD 26**
4 rounds
 1 minute plank
10 jump rope singles
1 minute plank (side)
10 jump rope singles
1 minute plank (other side)
10 jump rope singles
1 minute hollow hold
10 jump rope singles

**Jump Rope WOD 27**
30 rounds
50-25-5
 Double-unders
Thrusters
Front squats

**Jump Rope WOD 28**
For time
Row 1000m
60 Double-unders
10 HSPU
30 dips
30 push-ups
30 sit-ups
60x Double-unders

**Jump Rope WOD 29**
2 rounds for time
400m sprint
400 jump rope singles
50 pull-ups
50 double-unders

**Jump Rope WOD 30**
For time
100 double-unders

**Jump Rope WOD 31**
For time
50 unbroken jump rope singles
10 unbroken double-unders

**Jump Rope WOD 32**
5 rounds for time
20 pull ups
20 double-unders
20 jump rope singles

**Jump Rope WOD 33**
For time
100m sprint
100 double unders
20m bear crawl
20 jump rope singles
20 jumping jacks

**Jump Rope WOD 34**
2 rounds
20 HSPU
20 dips
20 goblet squats
20 unbroken double-unders

**Jump Rope WOD 35**

AMRAP in 9 minutes
3 deadlifts
3 muscle-ups
6 double-unders
12 jump rope singles

**Jump Rope WOD 36**

2 round for max reps
1 minute deadlifts
30 seconds Double unders
1 minute deadlifts
30 seconds Double unders
1 minute squats
1 minute jump rope singles

**Jump Rope WOD 37**

3 rounds
20 jump rope singles
20 push-ups
20 double-unders
20 push-ups

**Jump Rope WOD 38**
AMRAP in 20 minutes
5 snatches
10 pistols squats
15 double-unders

**Jump Rope WOD 39**
AMRAP in 15 minutes
5 L pull-ups
10 burpee broad jumps
15 jump rope singles

**Jump Rope WOD 40**
AMRAP in 10 minutes
6 squat clean
12 pull-ups
24 double-unders

**Jump Rope WOD 41**
25-10-5-4-3-2-1
squats
push-ups
sit-ups
Broad jumps
Toes to bar

## Jump Rope WOD 42
For time
25 Handstand push-ups
25 Double unders
55 KB swings
25 Double unders
25 Burpees
55 Push-ups
25 Pull-ups
25 Wall ball

## Jump Rope WOD 43
AMRAP in 13 minutes
7 pull-ups
50 wall ball shots
100 double-unders

## Jump Rope WOD 44
6 rounds
20 overhead press
5 power clean
25 double-unders

**Jump Rope WOD 45**

2 rounds

20 jump rope singles

20 double-unders

20 push-ups

20 sit-ups

20 pull-ups

20 squats

20 toes to bar

20 double-unders

20 jump rope singles

**Jump Rope WOD 46**

For time

100m sprint

 20 front squats

40 wall ball shots

60 burpees

80 double-unders

100m sprint

**Jump Rope WOD 47**
4 rounds
15 broad jumps
10 thrusters
20 jump rope singles
15 broad jumps
40 double-unders

**Jump Rope WOD 48**
2 rounds
50 walking lunges (25 per leg)
25 clean & press
50 jump rope singles
25 dips
50 wall ball shots
25 double-unders

**Jump Rope WOD 49**
AMRAP in 20 minutes
250m row
10 jump rope singles
100 push-ups
Row 250m

**Jump Rope WOD 50**
7 rounds for time
5 HSPU
10 deadlifts
10 pull-ups
5 double-unders

**Jump Rope WOD 51**
5 rounds
10 Double KB swing
12 toes to bar
14 double-unders

**Jump rope WOD 52**
For time
100 double unders
100 push-ups
100m sprint
100m bear crawl

**Jump Rope WOD 53**
AMRAP in 15 minutes
5 weighted pull-ups
10 thrusters
15 double-unders
25 jump rope singles

**Jump Rope WOD 54**
20-10-7
Push-ups
Jump rope singles
Sit-ups
Broad jumps
Pull-ups
Double-unders
Squats
Toes to bar

**Jump Rope WOD 55**
10 rounds for time
10 burpees
1 double under
10 sit-ups

## Jump Rope WOD 56

3 rounds for time

160m sprint

16 double-unders

160 jump rope singles

16 KB swings

## Jump Rope WOD 57

5 rounds

15 pull-ups

15 squats

15 box jumps

15 double-unders

15 push-ups

## Jump Rope WOD 58

AMRAP in 10 minutes

10 wall ball shots

10 power ssnatches

10 double unders

## Jump Rope WOD 59

AMRAP in 20 minutes

5 power cleans

10 pistol squats

15 double-unders

## Jump Rope WOD 60

AMRAP in 8 minutes

8 DB snatches (per arm)

8 toes to bar

8 double-unders

8 broad jumps

8 jump rope singles

**Jump Rope WOD 61**

2 rounds for time
100 double-unders
90 squats
80 sit-ups
70 push-ups
60 pull-ups
50 dips
40 box jumps
30 burpees
20 toes to bar
10 HSPU

**Jump Rope WOD 62**

3 rounds for time
10 double-unders
10 pull-ups
10 burpees
10 deadlifts
10 clean & press

## Jump Rope WOD 63

3 rounds
12 deadlifts
24 jump rope singles
6 double-unders
200m sprint

## Jump Rope WOD 64

5 rounds for time
10 burpees
15 walking lunges (per leg)
20 jump rope singles
100m sprint

## Jump Rope WOD 65

For time
Row 50 calories
100 jump rope singles
Row 40 calories
100 jump rope singles
Row 30 calories
100 jump rope singles
Row 20 calories
100 jump rope singles
Row 10 calories

**Jump Rope WOD 66**
3 rounds for time
30 double-unders
30 wall ball shots
30 broad jumps

**Jump Rope WOD 67**
50-40-30-20-10
Double-unders
Sit-ups
Push-ups
Jump rope singles

**Jump Rope WOD 68**
8 rounds for time
15 toes to bar
50 double-unders

**Jump Rope WOD 69**
2 rounds for time
400m sprint
15 HSPU
50 double-unders
25 jump rope singles

## Jump Rope WOD 70

4 rounds for time

100m sprint

10 jumping jacks

10 broad jumps

21 double-unders

10 KB renegade rows

5 push-ups

5 sit-ups

5 squats

# Kettlebell WODs

## KB WOD 1
EMOM for 12 minutes
1 KB clean
2 KB push press
3 KB push-ups

## KB WOD 2
4 rounds for time
21 double KB swing
21 double KB thruster
20 mountain climbers

## KB WOD 3
6 rounds for time
10 pistol squats (5 per leg)
10 box jumps
10 KB squats

## KB WOD 4
Max reps in 12 minutes
KB clean & jerk
KB is not to touch floor for duration of WOD

## KB WOD 5

AMRAP in 15 minutes

15 KB swings

15 KB squats

10 KB walking lunges (5 per leg)

## KB WOD 6

AMRAP in 20 minutes

3 KB pistol squats (per leg)

6 KB clean & press

9 KB snatch

## KB WOD 7

3 rounds for time

30 broad jumps

10 burpees

30 pull-ups

10 mountain climbers

30 push-ups

## KB WOD 8

2 rounds for time
80 KB swing
60 sit-ups
80 KB squats

## KB WOD 9

8 rounds
10 pistol squats (5 per leg)
1 minute plank
10 jumping jacks

## KB WOD 10

EMOM for 12 minutes
7 jumping jacks
7 burpees
7 push-ups

## KB WOD 11

AMRAP in 25 minutes

9 KB squats

10 push-ups

9 KB swings

10 push-ups

9 KB thrusters

10 push-ups

## KB WOD 12

For time

50 jumping jacks
50 KB deadlifts
50 burpees
50 KB squats

## KB WOD 13

AMRAP in 18 minutes
20 sit-ups
20 toes to bar
20 high knees
20 air squats
20 push-ups

## KB WOD 14

10 rounds for time
10 burpees
10 sit ups
10 jumping jacks
10 air squats
50m dash

## KB WOD 15

Tabata (8 intervals – 20 seconds work – 10 seconds rest)
KB swings
Pull-ups
KB squats
Jumping lunges

## KB WOD 16

4 rounds for time
12 KB thruster
12 sit-ups
20 KB push-ups
12 KB clean & jerk

## KB WOD 17

3 rounds for time
20 jump rope singles
20 diamond push-ups
20 KB swings

## KB WOD 18

EMOM for 20 minutes
1 burpee
2 KB thrusters
3 KB push-ups

**KB WOD 19**
For time
40 walking lunges (20 per leg)
10 KB snatches
10 KB push-ups
40 double KB squats

**KB WOD 20**
5 rounds
Max KB thrusters in 2 minutes
Max double KB squats in 2 minutes
Max KB push-ups in 2 minutes

**KB WOD 21**
5 rounds for time
10 pull-ups
10 KB snatches
10 KB swings
10 pistol squats

## KB WOD 22

21-15-9 for time

KB push-ups
Sit-ups
KB clean & jerk
KB walking lunges (per leg)

## KB WOD 23

50-40-30-20-10-5 for time

KB goblet squats
KB swings
One arm KB press

## KB WOD 24

50-40-30-20-10 reps

Squat jumps

Single KB thruster
KB sumo deadlift
KB farmers walk (reps = metres)

## KB WOD 25

EMOM for 14 minutes

3 KB deadlifts

3 KB clean & jerk

3 diamond push-ups

**KB WOD 26**

3 rounds for time
20 KB push-ups
50 KB goblet squats
21 KB sumo deadlifts
15 jumping jacks

**KB WOD 27**

EMOM for 15 minutes
5 air squats
6 KB walking lunges (per leg)
2 mountain climbers
1 KB deadlift

**KB WOD 28**

For time (partition as necessary)
100 pull-ups
100 push-ups
100 sit-ups
100 mountain climbers

**KB WOD 29**

AMRAP in 12 minutes
5 KB windmills
5 KB thrusters
5 KB clean & jerk

## KB WOD 30

22-11-8-4-2
KB front squat
KB clean & jerk
KB goblet squat
KB thrusters
Jumping jacks

# Rowing WODs

## ROWING WOD 1

Intervals
Row 4x1200m
Rest 2 minutes between intervals

## ROWING WOD 2

Time trial
Row 1500m
Damper setting at 10

## ROWING WOD 3

Intervals
Cover max distance
Row 6x[90:90]

## ROWING WOD 4

2 rounds
Rest for exact amount of time as previous row interval
Row 250m
Rest
Row 500m
Rest
Row 1000m
Rest
Row 2000m
Rest

## ROWING WOD 5

5 rounds
Rowing intervals, use total distance or calories as score
10:10
20:10
10:10
30:10
15:10
25:60

## ROWING WOD 6

Intervals
Row 10x250m
Rest 1 minute between intervals

## ROWING WOD 7

Intervals
Row 6x[90:90]

## ROWING WOD 8

Time trial
Cover max distance
Row 25 minutes

## ROWING WOD 9
Intervals
Rest 2 minutes between intervals
Row 6x500m

## ROWING WOD 10
Intervals
Cover max distance
Row 10x[60:60]

## ROWING WOD 11
Intervals
Cover max distance
Row 8x[30:20]

## ROWING WOD 12
Intervals
Cover max distance
Row 6x[90:90]

## ROWING WOD 13

For time
Row 50 calories
Rest 4 minutes
Row 40 calories
Rest 3 minutes
Row 30 calories
Rest 2 minutes
Row 20 calories
Rest 1 minute
Row 10 calories

## ROWING WOD 14

Intervals
Row 4x1200m
Rest 2 minutes between intervals

## ROWING WOD 15

Intervals
2 rounds, cover max distance
Row 1 minute
Rest 1 minute
Row 1 minute
Rest 50 seconds
Row 1 minute
Rest 40 seconds
Row 1 minute
Rest 30 seconds
Row 1 minute
Rest 20 seconds
Row 1 minute
Rest 10 seconds

## ROWING WOD 16

Time trial
Cover max distance
Row 25 minutes

## ROWING WOD 17

Tabata
Cover max distance possible
Row 8x[20:10]

## ROWING WOD 18

Intervals
Cover max distance during each interval
Row 3 minutes
Rest 2 minutes
Row 3 minutes
Rest 3 minute
Row 3 minutes
Rest 1 minute
Row 3 minutes
Rest 3 minute
Row 3 minutes
Rest 1 minute

## ROWING WOD 19

Intervals
2 rounds, cover max distance
Row 1 minute
Rest 1 minute
Row 1 minute
Rest 50 seconds
Row 1 minute
Rest 40 seconds
Row 1 minute
Rest 30 seconds
Row 1 minute
Rest 20 seconds
Row 1 minute
Rest 10 seconds

## ROWING WOD 20
Intervals
Rest 45 seconds between intervals
Row 8x250m

## ROWING WOD 21
Intervals
Rest 2 minutes between intervals
Row 6x500m

## ROWING WOD 22
Intervals
Row 10x250m
Rest 1 minute between intervals

## ROWING WOD 23
Tabata
Cover max distance possible
Row 8x[20:10]

## ROWING WOD 24
Time trial
Cover max distance
Row 10 min

## ROWING WOD 25
Time trial
Cover max distance
Row 10 min

## ROWING WOD 26
Intervals
Rest 45 seconds between intervals
Row 8x250m

## ROWING WOD 27
Intervals
Rest 2 minutes between intervals
Row 6x500m

## ROWING WOD 28
Intervals
Cover max distance during each interval
Row 3 minutes
Rest 1 minute
Row 3 minutes
Rest 3 minute
Row 3 minutes
Rest 1 minute
Row 3 minutes
Rest 3 minute
Row 3 minutes

## ROWING WOD 29
Intervals
Row 4x1200m
Rest 2 minutes between intervals

## ROWING WOD 30
Intervals
Row 20x[15:10]

## ROWING WOD 31
Intervals
Row 4x1200m
Rest 2 minutes between intervals

## ROWING WOD 32
Intervals
Row 20x[15:10]

## ROWING WOD 33
Intervals
For max distance
Row 20x[15:10]

## ROWING WOD 34
Rowing ladder
For total distance
Row 1 minute ON 1 minute OFF
Row 1 minute ON 50 seconds OFF
Row 1 minute ON 40 seconds OFF
Row 1 minute ON 30 seconds OFF
Continue down ladder until 1 minute ON 10 seconds OFF
Proceed back up and finish with 1 minute ON 50 seconds OFF

## ROWING WOD 35
3 rounds
Row 500m
Row 200m, upper body only
Rest 1 minute

## ROWING WOD 36
Intervals
Cover max distance
Row 8x[30:20]

## ROWING WOD 37
Intervals
Rest 2 minutes between intervals
Row 6x500m

## ROWING WOD 38
5 rounds
Partner effort, one rows while the other rests, switch until all rounds done
Row 50-40-30-20-10 calories

## ROWING WOD 39
3 rounds
Total calories = score
Row 2 minutes
Rest 3 minutes
Row 1 minute, arms only
Rest 1 minute
Row 1 minute
Rest 3 minutes

## ROWING WOD 40
Intervals
Rest 2 minutes between intervals
Row 6x500m

## ROWING WOD 41
Time trial
Row 8000m

## ROWING WOD 42
Intervals
Record average time for all intervals, this is an all out effort.
Row 10x250m
Rest for 5x(interval time) after each row interval

## ROWING WOD 43
Intervals
Rest 2 minutes between intervals
Row 6x500m

## ROWING WOD 44
Intervals
Row 4x1200m
Rest 2 minutes between intervals

## ROWING WOD 45
Tabata
Cover max distance possible
Row 8x[20:10]

## ROWING WOD 46
Time trial
Row 1500m
Damper setting at 10

## ROWING WOD 47

Intervals
2 rounds, cover max distance
Row 1 minute
Rest 1 minute
Row 1 minute
Rest 50 seconds
Row 1 minute
Rest 40 seconds
Row 1 minute
Rest 30 seconds
Row 1 minute
Rest 20 seconds
Row 1 minute
Rest 10 seconds

## ROWING WOD 48

Intervals
Record average time for all intervals
Row 10x250m
Rest for 5x(interval time)

## ROWING WOD 49

Intervals
Cover max distance
Row 10x[60:60]

## ROWING WOD 50

For time
Row 5K
500x reps of any combination of abdominal exercises

## ROWING WOD 51

Time trial
Row 4000m

## ROWING WOD 52

Intervals
2 rounds, cover max distance
Row 1 minute
Rest 1 minute
Row 1 minute
Rest 50 seconds
Row 1 minute
Rest 40 seconds
Row 1 minute
Rest 30 seconds
Row 1 minute
Rest 20 seconds
Row 1 minute
Rest 10 seconds

## ROWING WOD 53
Intervals
Record average time for all intervals, this is an all out effort.
Row 10x250m
Rest for 5x(interval time) after each row interval

## ROWING WOD 54
Intervals
Rest exactly 2 minutes between intervals, cover max distance possible
Row 4x8 minutes

## ROWING WOD 55
For time
Row 50 calories
Rest 4 minutes
Row 40 calories
Rest 3 minutes
Row 30 calories
Rest 2 minutes
Row 20 calories
Rest 1 minute
Row 10 calories

## ROWING WOD 56

4 rounds for max distance
Row 2 minutes
Rest 1 minute

## ROWING WOD 57

3 Rounds For Reps:
1 Minute Wall Ball Shots (20# / 14#)
1 Minute SDHP (75# / 55#)
1 Minute Box Jumps (20 / 20)
1 Minute Push Presses (75# / 55#)
1 Minute Row
1 Minute Rest
One point is given for each rep, except on the rower, where each calorie is one point.

## ROWING WOD 58

AMRAP 10 Minutes:
10 Calorie Row
10 Burpees

## ROWING WOD 59

In teams of 2
For Time:
5,000 Mete Row
Only one athlete can be working at a time.

## ROWING WOD 60

For Time:
400/40/4, 300/30/3, 200/20/2, 100,10,1
Row
Air Squats
Rope Climbs (15\')

## ROWING WOD 61

5 Rounds For Time:
5 Squats (275# / 205#)
500 Meter Row
Rest as needed between rounds.

## ROWING WOD 62

4 Rounds For Time:
250 Meter Row
AMRAP Burpee Pull-ups

## ROWING WOD 63

3 Rounds For Reps:
1 Minute Wall Ball Shots (20# / 14#)
1 Minute SDHP (75# / 55#)
1 Minute Box Jumps (20 / 20)
1 Minute Push Presses (75# / 55#)
1 Minute Row
1 Minute Rest
One point is given for each rep, except on the rower, where each calorie is one point.

## ROWING WOD 64

AMRAP 12 Minutes:
12 Calorie Row
12 Burpees

## ROWING WOD 65

AMRAP 30 Minutes:
1000 Meter Row
10 Wall Climbs

## ROWING WOD 66

For Time:
21-15-9
KB Swings (2 Pood / 1.5 Pood)
Row (calories)

## ROWING WOD 67

3 Rounds For Time:
1,000 Mete Row
50 Burpees
50 Box Jumps (24" / 20")
800 Meter Run

## ROWING WOD 68
Tabata
Row
Air Squats
Pull-ups
Push-ups
Sit-ups

## ROWING WOD 69
3 Rounds For Time:
1000 Meter Row
Each row will be max effort.
Rest as long as needed between rounds.
Score will be total time.

## ROWING WOD 70

In teams of 2
AMRAP 12 Minutes
12 Calorie Row
12 Burpees
One athlete will row while the other completes the burpees.
Athletes will switch stations and begin the next round, only after both athletes have completed their reps.

## ROWING WOD 70

5 Rounds For Time:
5 Squats (275# / 205#)
500 Meter Row
Rest as needed between rounds.

## ROWING WOD 71

For Time:
30 Pull-ups
20 Row (calories)
10 Deadlifts (275# / 205#)
10 Handstand Push-ups
20 Ring Dips
30 Burpees

## ROWING WOD 72

6 Rounds for Reps:
1 Minute Row
1 Minute Burpees
1 Minute Double-unders
1 Minute Rest
Score each exercise separately, as well as total.
Row is for calories.

## ROWING WOD 73

AMRAP 10 Minutes:
10 Calorie Row
10 Burpees

## ROWING WOD 74

5 Rounds For Time:
500 Meter Row
Each row will be max effort.
Rest as long as needed between rounds.
Score will be total time.

## ROWING WOD 75

Tabata
Wall Ball Shots (20# / 14#)
SDHP (75# / 55#)
Box Jumps (20 / 16)
Push Presses (75# / 55#)
Row (calories)
Score is total reps.

## ROWING WOD 76

For Time:
21-15-9
KB Swings (2 Pood / 1.5 Pood)
Row (calories)

## ROWING WOD 77

Tabata
Row (calories)
Air Squats
Pull-ups
Push-ups
Sit-ups
Rest one minute after each Tabata cycle. Tabata score is the least number of reps performed in any of the eight intervals.

## ROWING WOD 78

AMRAP 14 Minutes:
60 Calorie Row
50 Toes-to-bars
40 Wall Ball Shots (20# / 14#)
30 Cleans (135# / 95#)
20 Muscle-ups

## ROWING WOD 79

AMRAP 12 Minutes:
12 Calorie Row
12 Burpees

## ROWING WOD 80

AMRAP 20 Minutes
5 Power Cleans (95# / 65#)
5 Front Squats (95# / 65#)
5 Push Presses (95# / 65#)
500 Meter Row

# Running WODs

## Running WOD 1
AMRAP in 14 minutes
10 push-ups
10 ring pull-ups
100m sprint

## Running WOD 2
For time
Sprint 100m
83 OH walking lunges
70 squats
83 reverse OH walking lunge steps
35 push-press
Sprint 100m
15 thrusters
83 walking lunge steps
35 burpees
83 reverse walking lunge steps
35 wall ball
Sprint 100m
70 double unders
Sprint 100m

## Running WOD 3

2 rounds
 20 broad jumps
30 Double KB press
20 squats
30 KB renegade rows
Sprint 100m
20 KB swings
30x Double KB front squat
20 KB snatch
Sprint 100m
30 pull-ups
20 sit-ups
30 push-ups
Sprint 100m
20 broad jumps

## Running WOD 4

6 rounds for time
Sprint 100m
 1 minute max reps deadlift (1.5 bodyweight)
Sprint 100m

**Running WOD 5**

3 rounds
10 front squat
Sprint 100m
15 pull-ups
Sprint 100m
10 burpees

**Running WOD 6**

For time
Row 20 calories
Sprint 100m
Row 30 calories
Sprint 100m
Row 40 calories
Sprint 100m
Row 50 calories
Sprint 100m
Row 60 calories

**Running WOD 7**

6 rounds for time
50m sprint
 50 skipping rope singles
15 box jumps
50m sprint

**Running WOD 8**

Max rounds in 12 minutes
 10 push-press
Sprint 200m

**Running WOD 9**

For time
 Row 800m
7 pull-ups
14 KB swings
17 box jumps
14 burpees
7 sprint lunges
30 push-ups
40 flutter kicks
40 squats

## Running WOD 10
8 rounds
 Deadlift 6-12-18
Thruster 6-12-18
100m sprint

## Running WOD 11
4 rounds
 Thrusters 15-12-9-5
Sprint 100m
Deadlifts 15-12-9-5
Sprint 100m

## Running WOD 12
2 rounds
14 deadlifts
50m sprint
14 pistol squats
28 bodyweight squats
50m sprint

**Running WOD 12**
6 rounds
20 KB swing
100m sprint
10 burpees
100m sprint

**Running WOD 13**
5 rounds
5 hang power cleans
50m sprint
50m bear crawl

**Running WOD 14**
For time
Row 50 calories
Sprint 100m
Row 40 calories
Sprint 100m
Row 30 calories
Sprint 100m
Row 20 calories
Sprint 100m
Row 10 calories
Sprint 100m

### Running WOD 15
7 rounds
7 thrusters
70m sprint
17 pull-ups

### Running WOD 16
5 rounds
15 KB swing
15 Double KB snatch
30 squats
150m sprint

### Running WOD 17
10 rounds
100m sprint
10 pull-ups
10 burpees
100m sprint

### Running WOD 18
5 rounds
Sprint 100m
18 walking lunges (9 per leg)
9 burpees

**Running WOD 19**

8 rounds
 Sprint 100m
8x KB swings (72#)
5x Pull-ups, strict

**Running WOD 20**

4 rounds
 20 pull-ups
20 push-ups
50m sprint
20 KB swings
20 deadlifts

**Running WOD 21**

For time
Row 100 calories
Sprint 100m
Row 100 calories
Sprint 100m
Row 100 calories
Sprint 100m
Row 100 calories
Sprint 100m
Row 100 calories
Sprint 100m

**Running WOD 22**

AMRAP in 15 minutes
20 burpees
100m sprint
15 pull-ups
50m sprint

**Running WOD 23**

25 rounds
5 burpees
50m sprint

**Running WOD 24**

5 rounds
100m sprint
10 DB power snatch
10 DB overhead squats
100m sprint

**Running WOD 25**

3 rounds for time
Sprint 100m
20 burpees
20 DB push press
20 Squats
20 KB swings
Sprint 100m
20x Double KB front squats
20 KB snatch
20 push-ups
Sprint 100m

**Running WOD 26**
8 rounds
 4 deadlift

40m sprint
14 clapping push-ups
4 burpees

**Running WOD 27**
Max reps in 10 minutes
15 thrusters
Sprint 40m
15 thrusters
Sprint 40m
Max pull-ups

**Running WOD 28**
10 rounds
 10m Walking handstand
Sprint 50m between each set

## Running WOD 29
3 rounds
50m sprint
30 ball slams
30 box jumps
100m sprint

## Running WOD 30
AMRAP in 12 minutes
10m sprint
10 push-ups
20m sprint
20 sit-ups

## Running WOD 31
Holbrook
10 rounds for time
5 thrusters
10 pull-ups
100m sprint

**Running WOD 32**

8 rounds

12 push-ups

12 hollow rocks

100m sprint

**Running WOD 33**

5 rounds for time

10 tuck jumps

100m run

20 tuck jumps

200m run

**Running WOD 34**

For time

200m run

20 pull-ups

200m run

20 pull-ups

100m run

10 pull-ups

## Running WOD 35
3 rounds for time
400m run
15 power cleans
30 double-unders

## Running WOD 36
AMRAP in 14 minutes
20 deadlifts
400m sprint

## Running WOD 37
For time
600m run
20 KB swings
20 pull-ups
20 KB swings
2- push-ups
600m run

## Running WOD 38
AMRAP in 15 minutes
8 snatches
8 push-ups
300m sprint

**Running WOD 39**
AMRAP in 15 minutes
400m run
5 pull-ups
10 HSPU

**Running WOD 40**
7 rounds for time
12 deadlift
12 wall ball
200m sprint

**Running WOD 41**
AMRAP in 10 minutes
3 cleans
20 sit-ups
200m run

**Running WOD 42**
4 rounds for time
12 power cleans
200m sprint

### Running WOD 43
AMRAP in 21 minutes

400m sprint

20 air squats

10 broad jumps

### Running WOD 44
13 rounds for time

100m run

10 KB swings

10 toes to bar

### Running WOD 45
10 rounds

150m run

8 pull-ups

7 squats

7 burpees

### Running WOD 46
10 rounds

15 cleans

50m sprint

**Running WOD 47**
AMRAP in 20 minutes
2 Snatches
20 Sit-ups
200m run

**Running WOD 48**
For time
30 clean and press
100m sprint
10 burpees
300m sprint
10 broad jumps

**Running WOD 49**
7 rounds
10 deadlifts
100m sprint
50 double-unders
50m sprint

**Running WOD 50**

AMRAP in 20 minutes

300m sprint

5 pull-ups

5 HSPU

**Running WOD 51**

For time

800m run

50 push-ups

100 power clean s

100 sit-ups

800m run

**Running WOD 52**

5 rounds

10 front squats

50m dash

10 deadlifts

50m dash

## Running WOD 53

For time

30 sumo deadlift

300m sprint

25 snatch

300m sprint

25x clean and press

300m sprint

25 deadlifts

## Running WOD 54

5 rounds

20m sprint

8 KB swings

40m sprint

16 push-ups

60m sprint

24 sit-ups

**Running WOD 55**

3 rounds
200m sprint
20 second rest
400m sprint
40 second rest
600m sprint
60 second rest

**Running WOD 56**

For time
300m sprint
30 push-ups
10 snatches

**Running WOD 57**

AMRAP in 15 minutes
700m row
7 squats
7 pull-ups
20 push-ups
100m sprint

**Running WOD 58**

3 rounds for time
300m sprint
20 thrusters
10 burpees

**Running WOD 59**

For time
400m sprint
30x double KB snatch
300m sprint
30x KB clean and jerk
300m sprint
30x KB shoulder press
400m sprint

**Running WOD 60**

8 rounds
400m sprint
30x sit-ups
10x pull-ups
50m dash

## Running WOD 61
6 rounds
Run 800m
5 push-ups
5 sit-ups
5 squats

## Running WOD 62
For time
600m sprint
20 pull-ups
30 box jumps
20 double-unders
50 air squats
200m sprint
20 toes to bar
400m sprint

## Running WOD 63
3 rounds
20 squat cleans
20 burpees
200m sprint

**Running WOD 64**

5 rounds for time
200m sprint with weighted vest
20 wall balls
10 box jumps
10 overhead squats

**Running WOD 65**

2 rounds for time
 30 pull-ups
400m sprint
15 pull-ups
800m sprint
8 pull-ups

**Running WOD 66**

AMRAP in 17 minutes
400m sprint
5 pull-ups
10 push-ups
400m sprint
20 sit-ups
20 box jumps

**Running WOD 67**
For time
 300m sprint
40 squats
10 pull-ups
40 push-ups
800m sprint

**Running WOD 68**
4 rounds for time
 Run 200m
50 air squats
Run 300m
50 overhead squats
Run 100m
50 goblet squats
Run 50m

**Running WOD 69**
For time
800m run
400m backwards run
800m run
400m backwards run

## Running WOD 70

1km run stopping every 100m to perform 10 push-ups, 10 sit-ups and 10 squats

# Swimming WODs

## Swimming WOD 1

For max distance

Swim 8 intervals of 20 seconds on, 10 seconds off

Tread water during 10 second intervals

## Swimming WOD 2

For time

50m KB farmers carry underwater

200m Underwater dolphin kick with fins

500x Double-unders

50m KB farmers carry underwater

Swim 100m freestyle

Swim 100m backstroke

## Swimming WOD 3

For time

Swim 500m style of choice

Paddle 2000m

Swim 500m style of choice (different to previous)

**Swimming WOD 4**

AMRAP in 20 minutes

20x/arm KB push press

20x KB Goblet squat

10x/arm KB snatch

25m underwater KB carry

**Swimming WOD 5**

10 rounds for time

Swim 15m underwater

Swim 35m

Kick back 35m

Rest 1 minute

**Swimming WOD 6**

3 rounds for time

Swim 100m

30x KB swings

30x body rows

Swim 100m

**Swimming WOD 7**

6 rounds
Swim 25m
25x Squats
Swim 25m underwater
25x KB swings
Tread water for 2 minutes
Rest 1 minute

**Swimming WOD 8**

4 rounds for time
Swim 200m
25x Wall balls
30x Push-ups
Swim 200m
10x sit-ups

**Swimming WOD 9**

3 rounds for time
Swim 200m
30x KB swings
Swim 100m
30x Pull-ups
Swim 50m

**Swimming WOD 10**
2 rounds for time
30x Pull-ups
Swim 50m backstroke
30x Push-ups
Swim 50m butterfly
60x Sit ups
Swim 50m freestyle

**Swimming WOD 11**
6 rounds
Swim 100m
25x Pull-ups
Swim 100m
25x Push-ups

**Swimming WOD 12**
2 rounds
Swim 50m
50-40-30x Power clean
Swim 25m underwater
10 bodyweight squats
Rest 1 minute

## Swimming WOD 13
4 rounds
Swim 25m
25x Squats
Swim 25m
40x KB swings
Rest 1 minute

## Swimming WOD 14
3 rounds
20x man-makers
Swim 100m
10x/arm KB snatch
20x deadlifts
Swim 100m

## Swimming WOD 15
3 rounds
45lb plate roll 25m underwater
Swim 50m
45lb plate roll 25m underwater
Swim 50m
45lb plate roll 25m underwater
Swim 50m
Rest 3 minutes

**Swimming WOD 16**
For max distance
Swim 5x 30 seconds on, 15 seconds off
Tread water during 15 second rest interval

**Swimming WOD 17**
AMRAP in 20 minutes
25m KB farmers carry underwater
25 Push-ups
Swim 50m

**Swimming WOD 18**
For time
100 squats
Swim 100m freestyle
Swim 50m backstroke
Swim 25m underwater
Swim 25m underwater
100 squats

## Swimming WOD 19
AMRAP in 15 minutes
Swim 25m
25 push-ups
25 sit-ups
Swim 25m

## Swimming WOD 20
7 rounds for time
Swim 50m
10x Handstand push-ups
Swim 50m
10x Poolside get-outs
Rest 1 minute

## Swimming WOD 21
For max reps
Tread water 3 minutes
1 minute push-ups
Tread water 2 minutes
1 minute sit-ups
Tread water 1 minute
1 minute squats
Tread water 30 seconds
30 seconds burpees

**Swimming WOD 22**
5 rounds
Underwater swim 25m
50x Squats

**Swimming WOD 23**
AMRAP in 15 minutes
Swim 100m
25x Burpees

**Swimming WOD 24**
AMRAP in 15 minutes
Swim 50m
2x Handstand push-ups
Add 2 additional HSPU for each additional round (e.g. 4, 6, 8 etc.)

**Swimming WOD 25**
3 rounds
10x Burpees
Swim 25m
25x Push-ups
Swim 25m underwater
5x deadlifts

**Swimming WOD 26**

10 rounds

Swim 25m underwater

Rest 1 minute

Every breath taken during swim is penalty of 20x push-ups

**Swimming WOD 27**

3 rounds

Swim 50m freestyle

Swim 50m underwater

20 burpees

20 push-ups

20 sit-ups

**Swimming WOD 28**

For time

50m Single KB farmers carry poolside

Swim 50m

100m Farmers Carry

Swim 100m

150m Farmers Carry

Swim 150m

10 push-ups

10 sit-ups

10 squats

**Swimming WOD 29**

4 rounds for time

15x KB snatch, right arm

30m one arm swim, left arm

15x KB snatch, left arm

30m one arm swim, right arm

Rest 2 minutes

**Swimming WOD 30**

5 rounds for time

10 KB clean & jerk per arm

Swim 50m

Rest 1 minute

**Swimming WOD 31**

5 rounds
25 Double-unders
25m swim

**Swimming WOD 32**

For time
Swim 600m
Paddle 200m
Swim 600m
Paddle 200m

**Swimming WOD 33**

9 rounds
100m freestyle
50x Squats
50m freestyle
100x push ups
Rest 3 minutes

**Swimming WOD 34**
AMRAP in 25 minutes
Swim 50m
50x Squats
Swim 50m
50x Sit-ups
Swim 50m
50x Push-ups
Swim 50m

**Swimming WOD 35**
For time
25m KB farmers walk underwater
100x Double-unders
Swim 100m
25m KB farmers walk underwater
100x Double-unders

**Swimming WOD 36**
4 rounds for time
10x Deadlift
Swim 25m backstroke
Swim 25m underwater
30x Push-ups
Tread water for 1 minute

**Swimming WOD 37**

3 rounds
Swim 100m
30x KB swings
30x burpees
Swim 100m

**Swimming WOD 38**

2 rounds
21x Deadlift
Swim 200m
21x Push-ups
Swim 200m
Rest 3 minutes

**Swimming WOD 39**

Wear fins and snorkel
5 rounds
Swim 200m
20x Sit-ups
25x Push-ups
35x Squats

**Swimming WOD 40**

AMRAP in 21 minutes
25m KB farmers walk underwater
100x Double-unders
25m KB farmers walk underwater
Swim 100m
100x Double-unders

**Swimming WOD 41**

4 rounds for time
200m swim
21 Dumbbell Squat Cleans
100m swim
5 burpees

**Swimming WOD 42**

For Time
Teams of 2
20lb underwater carry – 30m
50 squats with wall ball
25 Push-ups
20lb underwater carry – 30m

**Swimming WOD 43**

5 rounds for time

25m swim

25 Thrusters

25m underwater swim

25 push-ups

**Swimming WOD 44**

AMRAP in 20 minutes

Swim 50m

25 Push-ups

25 Squats

Swim 50m

25 Double-Unders

Swim 50m

**Swimming WOD 45**

6 rounds for time

20m swim

50 bodyweight squats

20m underwater swim

20 burpees

**Swimming WOD 46**

AMRAP in 17 minutes

Swim 200m

30 Kettlebell swings

30 Pull-ups

Swim 200m

**Swimming WOD 47**

4 rounds for time

Swim 100m

25 DB push-press

Swim 100m

25 DB thrusters

**Swimming WOD 48**

AMRAP in 17 minutes

Swim 300m

25 Dumbbell Thrusters

Swim 150m

25 Goblet squats

## Swimming WOD 49
5 rounds for time
Swim 50m
25 push-ups
Swim 25m
50 push-ups

## Swimming WOD 50
For time
100m Swim
20 push-ups
20 sit-ups
20 squat
100m swim

## Swimming WOD 51
4 Rounds for time
10 push-ups
20m swim
30 squats
40 sit-ups
50m swim

**Swimming WOD 52**

100m swim

15 squats

15 push-ups

100m Swim

**Swimming WOD 53**

2 rounds for time

40 push-ups

swim 50m

40 squats

Swim 50m

30 push-ups

Swim 50m

30 Squat

**Swimming WOD 54**

AMRAP in 25 minutes

Swim 50m

50 push-ups

swim 25m underwater

20 walking lunges (per leg)

## Swimming WOD 55

For time

100m swim

100 push ups

100 squats

50m swim

50 push ups

50 squats

50m swim

1 minute plank

## Swimming WOD 56

20 squats

200m swim

50 push-ups

500m swim

25 burpees

250m swim

**Swimming WOD 57**

5 rounds for time

20 squat jumps

20 push-ups

20m swim underwater

30 second treading water

10 pool muscle-ups

**Swimming WOD 58**

4 rounds for time

50m swim

20 deadlifts

15 push-ups

50m swim underwater

20 deadlifts

50m backstroke swim

**Swimming WOD 59**

AMRAP in 14 minutes

50m backstroke

20 deadlifts

50m freestyle

20 push-ups

Tread water for 1 minute

20 push-ups

**Swimming WOD 60**

6 rounds for time

20m swim

20 bodyweight squats

20m swim

20 burpees

20m swim

20 push-ups

20 walking lunges (per leg)

Tread water for 1 minute

# Wall Ball WODs

## Wall Ball WOD 1
AMRAP in 20 minutes
8 hanging power cleans
12 wall ball shots
200m sprint
12 wall ball shots

## Wall Ball WOD 2
7 rounds for time
10 wall ball shots
5 burpees
12 wall ball shots
7 burpees
14 wall ball shots
9 burpees

## Wall Ball WOD 3
AMRAP in 10 minutes
5 wall ball shots
3 HSPU
1 power clean

## Wall Ball WOD 4
8 rounds for time
5 push-ups
5 pull-ups
10 wall ball shots

## Wall Ball WOD 5
AMRAP in 25 minutes
5 power cleans
15 wall ball shots
10 toes to bar
15 wall ball shots

## Wall Ball WOD 6
3 rounds for time
150 wall ball shots
75 double-unders
30 pull-ups

## Wall Ball WOD 7

For time

50 wall ball shots

50 box jumps

50 pull-ups

50 KB swings

50 walking lunges

50 toes to bar

50 clean and press

50 wall ball shots

50 wall ball shots

## Wall Ball WOD 8

For time

120 wall ball shots

## Wall Ball WOD 9

AMRAP in 12 minutes

21-15-9

Wall Ball Shots

Push-ups

Burpees

## Wall Ball WOD 10

10 rounds for time
5 pull-ups
5 push-ups
10 wall ball shots

## Wall Ball WOD 11

AMRAP in 5 minutes
5 wall ball shots
3 HSPU
1 deadlift

## Wall Ball WOD 12

6 rounds for time
3 power cleans
9 burpees
6 wall ball shots

## Wall Ball WOD 13
For time
200m sprint
20 pull-ups
20 wall ball shots
200m sprint
20 pull-ups
20 wall ball shots
200m sprint
10 pull-ups
20 wall ball shots
200m sprint

## Wall Ball WOD 14
4 rounds for time
21 wall ball shots
21 box jumps
21 pull-ups

## Wall Ball WOD 15
AMRAP 12 Minutes
40 calorie row
40 wall ball shots

**Wall Ball WOD 16**

2 rounds

15 box jumps

15 Pull-ups

15 KB swings

15 walking lunges

15 toes to bar

15 push press

15 back extensions

15 wall ball shots

15 burpees

**Wall Ball WOD 17**

AMRAP in 15 minutes

10 wall ball shots

10 burpees

100m sprint holding wall ball

10 wall ball shots

100m sprint holding wall ball

10 wall ball shots

## Wall Ball WOD 18

AMRAP in 10 minutes
50 wall ball shots
90 jump rope singles
30 pull-ups
50 wall ball shots

## Wall Ball WOD 19

3 rounds for max reps
1 Minute wall ball shots
1 Minute SDHP
1 Minute box jumps
1 Minute push press
1 Minute Rest

## Wall Ball WOD 20

4 rounds for time

16 KB swings

16 box jumps

160m sprint

16 burpees

16 wall ball shots

## Wall Ball WOD 21

2 rounds for time

10 toes to bar

10 box jumps

100 wall ball shots

## Wall Ball WOD 22

6 rounds for time

8 wall ball shots

8 pull-ups

8 box jumps

## Wall Ball WOD 23
4 rounds for time
30 wall ball shots
30 burpee broad jumps
600m row
30 wall ball shots

## Wall Ball WOD 24
For time
100 ball slams
100 wall ball shots

## Wall Ball WOD 25
For time
50-40-30-20-10-5-3-1
KB Swings
Wall Ball Shots
Box Jumps
Push-ups

## Wall Ball WOD 26
4 rounds
40 double-unders
40 wall ball shots
40m broad jumps

**Wall Ball WOD 27**

AMRAP in 12 minutes

40 calorie row

40 toes-to-bars

40 wall ball shots

40 cleans

40 push-ups

**Wall Ball WOD 28**

AMRAP in 25 minutes

20 wall ball shots

5 burpees

5 pull-ups

20 wall ball shots

**Wall Ball WOD 29**

3 rounds for time

100 walking lunges (50 per leg)

30 wall ball shots

30 box jumps

10 push-ups

## Wall Ball WOD 30
For time
21-15-9
HSPU
Wall ball shots

## Wall Ball WOD 31
3 rounds for time
24 deadlifts
24 box jumps
24 wall ball shots
24 box jumps
24 wall ball shots

## Wall Ball WOD 32
2 rounds for time
20 HSPU
20 pull-ups
20 push-ups
20 Wall ball
20 burpees
20 sit-ups
20 second plank

## Wall Ball WOD 33

AMRAP in 20 minutes
 20m dash
2 wall ball shots
20m dash
2 burpees
2 sit-ups
5 push-ups
6 walking lunges (3 per leg)

## Wall Ball WOD 34

AMRAP in 20 minutes
 20 wall ball shots
20 deadlifts
20 Ring dips

## Wall Ball WOD 35

20-10-5
 Wall ball shots
Sit-ups
Jump rope singles

## Wall Ball WOD 36
5 rounds
20 Wall ball
15 KB swings
20 burpees
20 Wall ball
50m walking lunges
20 push-ups
20 Wall ball

## Wall Ball WOD 37
For time
10 wall balls
10 burpees
100 bodyweight squats
10 wall balls
10 burpees

## Wall Ball WOD 38
For time
100mwalking lunges
100 sit-ups
100 wall ball shots
10 pull-ups
10 dips

## Wall Ball WOD 39

For time
Row 1000m
20 wall ball shots
Run 1000m
20 wall ball shots
Cycle 1000m

## Wall Ball WOD 40

2 rounds for time
20 high knees
20 wall ball shots
10 jumping Jacks
10 wall ball shots
10 push-ups
10 wall ball shots

## Wall Ball WOD 41

4 rounds
20 KB snatches (10 per arm)
20 wall ball shots
20 push-ups

## Wall Ball WOD 42

4 rounds
30 wall ball shots
30 power snatches

## Wall Ball WOD 43

21-15-9-5
Wall ball shots
Burpees
SDHP
Thrusters
Wall ball shots

## Wall Ball WOD 44

For time
21 wall ball shots
21 deadlifts
21 box jumps
21 wall ball shots
21 push-ups
21 box jumps
21 wall ball shots
21 clean and press
21 wall ball shots

## Wall Ball WOD 45

3 rounds
 10 clean and jerk
50 wall ball shots

## Wall Ball WOD 46

6 rounds
10 KB renegade rows
15 wall ball shots
20 pull-ups

## Wall Ball WOD 47

9 rounds for time
5 pull-ups
5 power cleans
50 wall ball shots
5 box jumps
5 push-ups

## Wall Ball WOD 48
For time
 30 wall ball shots
100 KB swings
30 push-ups
100 sit-ups
30 squats
100 wall ball shots

## Wall Ball WOD 49
2 rounds
800m row
100m farmers walk with KB
30x sit-ups
20x wall ball shots
800m row
15 burpees
30 sit-ups
20x wall ball shots

**Wall Ball WOD 50**

6 rounds
21-15-9-5
Burpee broad jumps
KB press
Sit-ups
Deadlifts
Wall balls

**Wall Ball WOD 51**

4 rounds
20 wall ball shots
15 push-ups
10 pistols
5 deadlifts

## Wall Ball WOD 52

2 rounds

40 wall ball shots

30 deadlifts

20 box jumps

10 pull-ups

40 sit-ups

30 pull-ups

20 box jumps

10 wall ball shots

## Wall Ball WOD 53

For time

1000m row

10 squats

1000m row

10 push-ups

1000m row

10 KB swings

1000m row

10 wall ball shots

1000m row

## Wall Ball WOD 54

3 rounds of run 800m + 30x wall ball (up to 20#/14#) + 30x box jumps (up to 24/20"), rest 2:00 between rounds

Pre-teen:

3 rounds of run 200m + 10x wall ball (up to 8#) + 30x box jumps (up to 16"), rest 2:00 between rounds

Kids:

3 rounds of run 100m + 10x wall ball (up to 6#) + 10x box jumps (up to 12"), rest 2:00 between rounds

## Wall Ball WOD 55

8 rounds for time

10 wall ball shots

10 push-ups

10 wall ball shots

10 sit-ups

10 wall ball shots

10 squats

## Wall Ball WOD 56

15 rounds
1 wall ball shot
2 walking lunges
3 wall ball shots
4 walking lunges
5 wall ball shots
6 walking lunges
7 wall ball shots
8 walking lunges
9 wall ball shots
10 walking lunges

## Wall Ball WOD 57

2 rounds
69 double-unders
69 wall ball shots
69 burpees
69 deadlifts

**Wall Ball WOD 58**

AMRAP in 15 minutes

15 push-ups

15 ring dips

15 wall ball shots

15 sit-ups

15 wall ball shots

**Wall Ball WOD 59**

3 rounds for time

Sprint 100m

20 thrusters

20 burpees

20 wall ball shots

Sprint 100m

**Wall Ball WOD 60**

6 rounds for tme

21 wall ball shots

21 burpees

## Wall Ball WOD 61

9 rounds for time
10 broad jumps
10 sit-ups
10 deadlifts
10 KB renegade rows
10 wall ball shots

## Wall Ball WOD 62

AMRAP in 20 minutes
5 pull-ups
5 push-ups
5 sit-ups
50 wall ball shots

## Wall Ball WOD 63

2 rounds for time
50 pistol squats
40 front squats
30 wall ball shots
20 goblet squats
19 wall ball shots

## Wall Ball WOD 64

3 rounds

300m row

30 wall ball shots

30 box jumps

30 jump rope singles

30 sit-ups

30 toes to bar

## Wall Ball WOD 65

For time

10 HSPU

10 deadlifts

10 broad jumps

10 pull-ups

10 wall ball shots

100m dash

## Wall Ball WOD 66

3 rounds for time

21 wall ball shots

21 KB swings

## Wall Ball WOD 68

For time

500m row

50 wall ball shots

500m row

50 wall ball shots

Row 500m

50 wall ball shots

## Wall Ball WOD 69

For time

1000m row

21 wall ball shots

100m sprint

100 sit-ups

1 minute plank

## Wall Ball WOD 70

20 rounds for time

1 push-up

1 wall ball shot

1 sit-up

1 wall ball shot

1 bodyweight squat

1 wall ball shot

# Warmup WODs

**Warmup WOD 1**

5 minute AMRAP

10 walking lunges

100m jog

5 inch worms

**Warmup WOD 2**

3 rounds (maintain a moderate pace)

5 pull-ups

10 bodyweight squats

100m jog

**Warmup WOD 3**

5 minute AMRAP

20 jump rope singles

20 box jumps

20 walking lunges (10 per leg)

**Warmup WOD 4**

30 seconds of pull-ups

30 seconds of sit-ups

30 seconds of bodyweight squats

30 seconds of push-ups

**Warmup WOD 5**

10 burpees
10 push-ups
100m jog

**Warmup WOD 6**

20 KB swings
20 walking lunges (10 per leg)
10 pull-ups

**Warmup WOD 7**

3 rounds
20 bodyweight squats
10 wall ball shots
200m jog

**Warmup WOD 8**

Spend 1 minute on each exercise
Bodyweight squats
Push-ups
Walking lunges
Sit-ups

**Warmup WOD 9**

2 rounds
Row 10 calories
30 jump rope singles
20 box jumps

**Warmup WOD 10**

20 wall ball shots
20 push-ups
10 KB swings
10 burpees

# Conclusion

I hope you enjoy the plethora of workouts the Cross Training WOD Bible 2.0 has to offer you, by following these workouts on a regular basis you'll develop not only a strong, flexible, functionally fit body that'll be ready to tackle any situation life throws at it but also an unbreakable mindset and confidence to match.

Whether you're looking to get a competitive advantage in your sport or just to increase your mobility, strength and health these workouts are the answer.

I hope you enjoyed reading this book as much as I enjoyed writing it.

Until next time,

*P.S*

Made in the USA
Middletown, DE
26 April 2016